CW00944926

Ketogenic Diet: F Recipes

16 Recipe Keto Cookbook (Sweet and

Savory Snacks)

by Liam Barnes

Copyright © 2016 by Liam Barnes - All rights reserved.

No part of this document may be reproduced in any form or by any means, including scanning, photocopying, or otherwise without prior written permission of the copyright holder.

Introduction

Are you having troubles following somewhat strict ketogenic diet regime? Altough very healthy low-carb, high-fat diet most of the time doesn't come across as particulary tasty and easy to manage, especially in this day and age when there is huge variety of sugary food temptations rich in carbohydrates.

Ketogenic diet is known to lower your blood sugar and (bad) cholesterol, it decreases your body fat percentage and what is most important: with transitionin into state of ketosis increases your energy leves, mental clarity and overall well-being. This cookbook provides you with 16 recipes of nutritious sweet and savory keto snacks - so called fat bombs - that are cheap, quick and easy-to-make. With these you will get a firm proof food tastiness is in no way questionable for keto avid followers.

Thank you for purchasing this book and I hope you enjoy the recipes. Bon apetite!

Liam Barnes

Table of Contents

Macadamia Madness

Ingredients:

- 10 tbsp coconut oil
- 5 tbsp unsweetened cocoa powder
- 2 packets (2g) granulated sweetener
- 3 tbsp coarsely chopped macadamia nuts
- Coarse sea salt

Preparation:

1. On stovetop melt coconut oil.

2. Add cocoa powder and granulated Stevia. Mix and remove from heat.

3. Spoon mixture into silicone candy molds until wells are 3/4 full.

4. Refrigerate in silicone molds until mixture thickens.

5. Sprinkle macadamia nuts into each well. Press down to distribute the nuts throughout the mixture.

6. Return silicone mold to refrigerator until completely hardened.

7. Once completely set, remove chocolates from silicone mold and place right side up on a dish or cupcake liner.

8. Let sit at room temperature until surface begins to glisten.

9. Sprinkle a pinch of course sea salt onto each chocolate fat bomb.

10. Serve or return to refrigerator for storage.

Lemon Cheescake Wonder

Ingredients:

- 1/4 cup melted coconut oil
- 4 tbs softened unsalted butter
- 1 tbsp finely grated lemon juice
- 2 tsps sweetener
- 4 oz cream cheese

Preparation:

1. Mix all ingredients together with a hand mixer until very smooth.

2. Pour into silicone molds.

3. Freeze until firm.

4. Sprinkle with lemon zest.

Ginger Majesty

Ingredients:

- 2,6 oz softened coconut butter
- 2,6 oz softened coconut oil
- 0.8 oz unsweetened shredded coconut
- 1 tsp granulated stevia or other low-carb sweetener
- 1/2 tsp powdered ginger

Preparation:

1. Mix all the ingredients in a pouring jug until the stevia is dissolved.

2. Pour into silicon moulds or ice cube trays.

3. Refrigerate for 10 minutes or more and serve.

Coco Tropic Thunder

Ingredients:

- 2, 6 oz softened coconut butter
- 26 oz melted coconut oil
- 0,8 oz finely shredded coconut
- 1 tsp granulated stevia or other low-carb sweetener

Instructions:

1. Mix all the ingredients in a pouring jug until stevia is dissolved.
2. Pour into ice cube trays or silicon moulds.
3. Refrigerate for 10 minutes and serve.

Lime Paradise

Ingredients:

- 1 stick unsalted butter

- 3/4 c. coconut oil
- 1 oz. unsweetened, shredded coconut
- zest of 2 small limes
- juice of 2 small limes
- 4 oz. cream cheese
- 1/4 c. coconut cream (kind with no added sugar)
- 1/4 tsp vanilla extract
- low carb sweetener of your choice

Preparation:

1. Soften cream cheese and set it aside.

2. Melt butter and coconut oil in a medium saucepan over medium heat. Add zest and lime juice and stir. Add coconut, vanilla extract, coconut cream and, lastly, soft cream cheese. Whip all ingredients until smooth and add a sweetener.

3. Spoon mixture into silicone moulds.

4. Freeze for at least 30 minutes and serve.

Super Pecan Brownies

Ingredients:

- 1 4 oz unsweetened chocolate
- 3/4 cup butter
- 1 1/2 cup stevia
- 3 eggs
- 1 tsp. vanilla extract
- 1 cup almond flour
- 1/2 cup chopped pecans

Preparation:

1. Melt the chocolate and butter.

2. Add the rest of the ingredients to the bowl and mix it until smooth.

3. Pour into a greased 8x8 dish and bake at 350 for 30 minutes. Serve.

Caramel Joy

Ingredients:

BOTTOM LAYER:
- 1 cup milk chocolate chips
- 1/4 cup butterscotch chips
- 1/4 cup creamy peanut butter

FILLING:
- 1/4 cup butter
- 1 cup white sugar
- 1/4 cup evaporated milk
- 1 1/2 cups marshmallow creme
- 1/4 cup creamy peanut butter
- 1 teaspoon vanilla extract
- 1 1/2 cups chopped salted peanuts

CARAMEL:
- 1 (14 ounce) package individually wrapped caramels, unwrapped
- 1/4 cup heavy cream

TOP LAYER:

- 1 cup milk chocolate chips
- 1/4 cup butterscotch chips
- 1/4 cup creamy peanut butter

Preparation:

1. Lightly grease a 9x13 inch dish.

2. Bottom layer: Combine 1 cup milk chocolate chips, 1/4 cup butterscotch chips and 1/4 cup creamy peanut butter in a saucepan over low heat. Cook and stir until melted and smooth. Spread evenly in prepared pan. Refrigerate until set.

3. Filling: melt butter in a heavy saucepan over medium-high heat. Add 1 cup sugar and 1/4 cup evaporated milk. Bring to a boil, and let boil 5 minutes. Remove from heat and stir in marshmallow creme, 1/4 cup peanut butter and vanilla. Fold in peanuts. Spread over bottom layer, return to refrigerator until set.

4. Caramel: combine caramels and cream in a medium saucepan over low heat. Cook and stir until melted and smooth. Spread over filling. Chill until set.

5. Top layer: In a small saucepan over low heat, combine 1/4 cup butterscotch chips, 1 cup milk chocolate chips,

and 1/4 cup peanut butter. Cook and stir until melted and smooth. Spread over caramel layer. Chill 1 hour before cutting into 1 inch squares and serve.

Almond King Bars

Ingredients:

CAROB/CHOCOLATE BASE:
- 1/2 cup coconut oil
- 1/2 cup almond butter
- 1/4 cup granulated sweetener or appropriate substitute
- 6 tbsp carob or cocoa powder
- 3 tbsp additional sweetener
- 1 tsp vanilla

COCONUT TOPPING:
- 1 2/3 cup unsweetened coconut flakes
- 7 tbsp coconut oil
- 1/3 cup granulated sweetener
- 1 1/2 tsp vanilla

- 1/4 tsp additional flavoring (optional. Almond or coconut are good choices.)
- 2 tsp arrowroot powder.
- Almonds halves or slices

Preparation:

1. Melt oil and nut/seed butter over low heat.
2. Stir in carob and granulated sweetener and combine thoroughly.
3. Mix in remaining ingredients except for vanilla. Continuously stir until it slightly thickens, then remove from heat.
4. Stir in the vanilla.
5. While you make the topping pour the mixture into pan and place in freezer to harden.
6. Melt oil in small pan and add coconut flakes then stir it.
7. Add remaining ingredients. Simmer and stir until it thickens a bit.
8. When the chocolate is hardened, gently smooth the coconut mixture on top.
9. Place slivered or whole almonds on top. Place bars back in the freezer until hardened.
10. Slice into squares of desired size and serve.

Ultimate Ice-Cream

Ingredients:

- 1/2 cup extra virgin coconut oil, room temperature
- 1/2 cup butter
- 4 large egg yolks
- 2 large eggs
- 1/4 cup powdered erythritol or other low-carb sweetener
- 1 cup coconut milk or heavy whipping cream
- 2 vanilla beans

Preparation:

1. Separate the egg yolks from egg whites. Butter and coconut oil ought to be softened at room temperatureas this makes it easier to bind it with the egg yolks.

2. Mix the butter, coconut oil, vanilla extract and powdered erythritol sweetener together.

3. Slowly add the egg yolks and whole eggs while blending one by one and mix it until smooth.

4. While blending add the coconut milk.

5. Scoop the mixture into the ice-cream maker and process.

6. Half way through, remove from the ice-cream maker. Use an immersion blender and pulse until smooth.

7. Return to the ice-cream maker and continue until your ice-cream is done.

8. Eat immediately or place in the freezer for 30-60 minutes for ice-cream to harden. Keep in the freezer in single-serving containers.

Pizza Time

Ingredients:

- 4 oz cream cheese
- 2 tbsp sundried tomato pesto
- 14 slices pepperoni
- 8 pitted Black Olives
- 2 tbsp chopped fresh basil
- Salt and Pepper to taste

Preparation:

1. Dice pepperoni and olives.

2. Combine cream cheese, pesto and basil.

3. Add pepperoni, olives and mix well.

4. Form into balls and garnish. Serve.

Sweet Choco Dreams

Ingredients:

- 1/2 cup unsweetened cocoa powder
- 1/2 cup salted butter
- 1/2 cup cream cheese
- 1 cup granulated sweetener of choice
- 4 large eggs
- 3 tsp vanilla extract
- 5 tbs coconut oil
- 1/2 tsp baking powder
- 1 tsp olive oil (for greasing the pan)

Preparation:

1. Preheat your oven to 450 F.

2. Put butter and cream cheese into a large microwavable bowl, microwave on high for 1,5 to 2 minutes or until butter and cream cheese melts/softens.

3. Mix melted butter and cream cheese with a large spoon.

4. Add sweetener, cocoa powder, and coconut oil to the butter and cream cheese. Mix thoroughly.

6. While mixing separately add vanilla extract, baking powder and eggs. Mix until smooth.

7. Pour the batter into the cooking pan and spread it evenly.

11. Put into oven and bake for 35-40 minutes on 450 F.

12.Let it cool at least 15 minutes, slice it and serve.

Ultimate Macaroons

Ingredients:

- 1/3 cup coconut butter
- 2 tbsp coconut oil
- 1/2 tsp vanilla
- juice from 1/2 lemon
- optional lemon zest

- 1/2 tsp honey

Preparation:

1. Mix it in a food processor or by hand.
2. Add 1/4 to 1/3 cup dried or desiccated coconut. Hand mix together.
3. Dollop onto plastic wrap or parchment paper and let in the refrigerator until firm. Serve.

Peppermint Mocha Freshness

Ingredients:

- 3/4 cup melted coconut butter
- 3 tbsp melted coconut oil
- 3 tbsp hemp seeds
- 1/4 tsp peppermint extract
- 2 tbsp organic cocoa powder
- 5-8 drops liquid stevia

Preparation:

1. Mix together melted coconut butter, 1 tbsp of coconut oil, hemp seeds and peppermint extract.
2. Pour into moulds about 3/4 the way. Refrigerate until firm. Stir together 2 tbsp of melted coconut oil, cocoa powder and stevia. Sprinkle on top of fat bombs.
3. Refrigerate until firm. Pop out of moulds and serve.

Crazy Maple Bacon

Ingredients:

- 8 oz cream cheese
- 1/2 cup butter 4 tsp bacon fat
- 4 tbsp coconut oil
- 1/4 cup sugar-free maple syrup or other low-carb sweetener
- 6 strips crispy bacon

Preparation:

1. Combine all ingredients except bacon.
2. Melt slowly in microwave until smooth and mostly liquid.
3. Pour into silicone moulds and add a bit of bacon crumbles into each mould.
3. Put molds in freezer until firm. Serve.

Coco-Cinnamon Marbles

Ingredients:

- 1 cup coconut butter
- 1 cup coconut milk
- 1 tsp vanilla extract
- 1/2 tsp nutmeg
- 1/2 tsp cinnamon
- 1 tsp stevia powder extract or other low corb sweetener
- 1 cup coconut shreds

Preparation:

1. Place a glass bowl over a sauce pan with a few inches of water in it.

2. Put all the ingredients except shredded coconut in a double boiler over medium heat. Mix the ingredients while they are melting.

3. Remove the bowl from the heat.

4. Place the bowl in the fridge until the mixture is hard enough to roll into balls.

5. Roll the contents into one inch balls and roll them through the coconut shreds.

6. Refrigerate for one hour and serve.

Orange Creamsicle Utopia

Ingredients:

- 1/2 cup Coconut Oil
- 1/2 cup heavy whipping cream
- 4 oz cream cheese
- 1 tsp orange extract

- 10 drops liquid stevia

Preparation:

1. Blend together all of the ingredients with immersion blender until smooth
2. In the process of mixing add orange extract and liquid stevia.
4.Pour the mixture into silicone and freeze for 2-3 hours.
5. Serve when solid.

Conclusion

If you enjoyed this cookbook and found it useful, I would be very grateful if you would leave a short review on Amazon's website. All your feedback really makes a difference and with your help I am able to make my product even better.

Thank you for all your support.

23240860R00016

Printed in Poland
by Amazon Fulfillment
Poland Sp. z o.o., Wrocław